The A - Z
of
Weight Management

A transformational alphabet to help
you shed weight and become the
person you are ready to be!

HAZEL NEWSOM CHT

BALBOA.PRESS
A DIVISION OF HAY HOUSE

Balboa Press books may be ordered through booksellers or by contacting:

Balboa Press
A Division of Hay House
1663 Liberty Drive
Bloomington, IN 47403
www.balboapress.com
844-682-1282

Because of the dynamic nature of the Internet, any web addresses or links contained in this book may have changed since publication and may no longer be valid. The views expressed in this work are solely those of the author and do not necessarily reflect the views of the publisher, and the publisher hereby disclaims any responsibility for them.

The author of this book does not dispense medical advice or prescribe the use of any technique as a form of treatment for physical, emotional, or medical problems without the advice of a physician, either directly or indirectly. The intent of the author is only to offer information of a general nature to help you in your quest for emotional and spiritual well-being. In the event you use any of the information in this book for yourself, which is your constitutional right, the author and the publisher assume no responsibility for your actions.

Any people depicted in stock imagery provided by Getty Images are models, and such images are being used for illustrative purposes only. Certain stock imagery © Getty Images.

Print information available on the last page.

ISBN: 978-1-9822-4773-7 (sc)
ISBN: 978-1-9822-4772-0 (hc)
ISBN: 978-1-9822-4774-4 (e)

Library of Congress Control Number: 2020908853

Balboa Press rev. date: 06/24/2020

To my son Richard and daughter Natalie
For your help and encouragement

Who are you? When you look in the mirror who do you see? Do you see the person you feel you are inside? Are you surprised? Is that really me, you may be asking yourself. Perhaps when you look in the mirror you see a body that is far bigger than that which you want, or feel you are really. So, what can you do about it?

Every decision you make defines you in some way. So, do you define yourself as a person who is overweight, with eating habits that are out of control, and accept that this is it for the rest of your life? Probably not. If you did you would not be reading this book. So, you know who you want to be, but it has always been a question of how to become that person. Now you can start to make choices to be the person you want to be. Life is about choices. You have made certain choices in the past. Are you now ready to make different choices, ones that will have different results?

How many times have you tried to shed weight, only to find that you have regained it once you have come off the diet? You've put the pounds back on, usually gaining even more pounds. How many times have you been frustrated to find that you cannot eat what others around you are eating? How many times has that led to a feeling of deprivation? "Too many," you may be saying.

Like many people, you may be concerned about your health, you may feel self-conscious and you may struggle with the everyday acts of putting on your shoes, reaching behind your back and even bending down to pick up something from the floor. Every day an inconvenience hits you as you go about your daily life.

Like many, you have perhaps looked outside yourself for the answers to your weight problem. You have gone on a diet, you have started going to a gym, only to find yourself unmotivated to continue. You then feel frustrated and powerless. There is an overwhelming sense of hopelessness.

I see clients every day for weight reduction. When I ask "What is your commitment to getting rid of your unwanted weight on a level of 1 – 10?" and the answer is an 8 or 9, I ask "What does the other 1 or 2 represent?" And the most common reply is "Well, I've been on so many diets and I've failed so often, that there is a part of me that is afraid I will fail with this one too." And my response is that they have not failed, they have merely tried something that hasn't worked for them. Now they are looking for a new mind-set.

What you will read about here is not about dieting; this is about a new mind-set, a new way of relating to food. People who come to me are trying something different, hypnosis, which is a whole new way of dealing with weight release. You will note that I use the words "release" or "shed", not "lose." Losing something is a negative and your subconscious will want to find it again, but releasing is positive and empowering. YOU have made the decision to let go of the weight that you no longer want and need. However, even with hypnosis one has, at times, to make conscious choices. That is "The Conscious Edge" and you will find suggestions in this A – Z of Weight Management to help you with your conscious choices.

I see two kinds of clients for weight release; some for damage control and some for prevention. The damage control clients are those who already have diabetes, heart problems, knee replacements etc. The prevention clients are overweight but have gotten away with it so far, and realize that they are walking a fine line. Unfortunately, I see more of the former than the latter. Usually people will try all the diets they can. They are dedicated to the diets, but once they achieve their goal the vast majority eventually regain all the weight they lost – and more! They come to me as a last resort.

So, ask yourself, what is it that you really want? If you want to be healthy and fit, in control of your life and your eating habits, know that this is possible, this is attainable. If you haven't achieved this so far, know that you have been taking a path that has not led you to where you want to be. You may have been working with the wrong tools or maybe there wasn't a roadmap to show you the way.

You have now decided to go in a different direction. You are on a different track. Think of yourself starting out on a journey – the journey of a lifetime. That's right, the journey of a lifetime. This is not a short ride to the nearest store. Think of yourself as a traveler on a train heading for your destination. Everyone wants to be on the express train and reach their destination of slenderness, health and vitality quickly and without stops. However, most of us take the commuter train, and although it stops at stations on the way, and is slower, it still reaches the destination. Suppose you choose to have a chocolate bar for example, think of that as getting off at a station. So, metaphorically you should enjoy the scenery and get back on the train, back on track, as soon as you are able. The train will not leave without you; you are the engineer, the conductor and the passenger because this is your train and you have a ticket to ride – always!

In this book I would like to offer some practical ideas and suggestions for changing your mind-set. Should you decide to incorporate hypnosis, this would reinforce your commitment to yourself, but you yourself can make the changes slowly and effectively, one by one, day by day.

ENJOY THE JOURNEY – ENJOY THE RIDE

"The journey of a thousand miles begins with one small step."

———

LAO TZU

A IS FOR ATTITUDE

What is your attitude towards letting go of the weight? Is it something that you would like to do but...? Do you see it as deprivation? A punishment for the years of overeating? Something you will have to struggle with? Perhaps an act of defiance at someone who wants you to lose the weight? The effect of a habit that you cannot change?

Well, now is the time to adjust your attitude. You are at the beginning of a journey... a journey to health and vitality. You *can* have a positive attitude about yourself and your ability to reach your goal of being slim, fit and healthy.

"There is little difference in people, but that little difference makes a big difference. The little difference is ATTITUDE. The big difference is whether it is positive or negative."

___

W. CLEMENT STONE

A **IS FOR AFFIRMATIONS**

Support yourself with positive affirmations. These can be said quietly to yourself or out loud. You may find some of your own that sound good to you.

- ✓ *I now find myself wanting only foods that contribute to my good health.*
- ✓ *I appreciate my body so I eat only foods that nourish it.*
- ✓ *I love, respect and care for my body.*
- ✓ *I am able to release all the weight I want easily and effortlessly.*
- ✓ *Every day I find it easier and easier to avoid overeating.*
- ✓ *I will always maintain a healthy mind and body.*
- ✓ *I find it easier and easier to have less food on my plate.*
- ✓ *I am safe, and it is safe to let go of my unwanted pounds.*
- ✓ *I go through each day choosing healthy, nutritious food.*
- ✓ *Because I choose good health, I pay attention to my body's needs.*
- ✓ *I deserve to be slender, fit and healthy.*
- ✓ *I am now changing negative eating patterns into positive eating patterns.*
- ✓ *I find it easy to make healthy food choices.*
- ✓ *I am willing to release any past experience or belief that may be stopping me from reaching my goal of shedding excess pounds of fat.*
- ✓ *Every day in every way I am getting better and better.*

A IS FOR ACCEPTANCE

Accept yourself for who you are right now. Yes, you want to be slimmer, fitter maybe, but recognize the value and worth you have in you at this very moment. Can you look in the mirror and say "You know, you look good today?" Or do you feel uncomfortable giving yourself praise?

If a friend were to walk through the door and looked great, you would probably have no problem telling him or her so. We find it so easy to see what is imperfect in ourselves and much harder to give credit to ourselves. So, accept yourself as you are at this time. At the same time, resolve that you are making a change and that change will be welcome as you release your weight. It is not about all or nothing. You may not want to stay at the weight you are now, but don't tell yourself that you will only be happy when you have reached your goal of being slim.

Suppose you are 200 lbs and it frustrates and upsets you. How realistic is it to feel that you will only be truly happy with yourself when you are 130 lbs? Surely you will feel pretty good when you are 175 or 150 lbs. Accept yourself at every level as your weight decreases and you journey towards your goal.

B IS FOR BELIEF

Do you really believe you can be slim, trim and fit? You had better believe it if you want it to happen. As the saying goes "if the subconscious mind can conceive it and believe it, it can achieve it." So, start believing!

Believe that you deserve to reach your goal. Believe that you can reach your goal. If you struggle with this you may want to engage the help of a professional. Hypnosis is one way of achieving this. With hypnosis, you can reach down and replace negative self-talk with positive reinforcement on a subconscious level, which is where all beliefs are stored. With hypnosis you can re-frame the negative thoughts into positive thoughts. If you feel that hypnosis is not for you, keep the belief that you do indeed deserve to be slim and healthy firmly in your mind anyway.

"

"What do I believe that
I deserve in this life?"

———

**ELIZABETH GILBERT,
EAT, PRAY, LOVE**

"

B IS FOR BALANCE

A life well lived is a life in balance. We start out in life finding our balance. When you were a baby you began to find your balance. You would try to walk and lose your balance. Did you stop there, and then not try again? No, of course not! If you had, you would not be walking today. Once you found your balance there was no stopping you. You were off to the races. However, finding your balance probably didn't happen overnight, but you were determined to do it. So, what is different about you and your life now? Why accept a loss of balance?

Balance is the natural order of things. When any aspect of our life is out of balance it creates dis-harmony, dis-ease. Balance brings harmony, peace and fulfillment. Look at where there is imbalance in your life. If it is in your eating habits, look at ways in which you can bring them back into balance with the rest of your life.

My life is in balance
I am in control

B IS FOR BODY

Love your body. It's the only one you get. You cannot trade it in for a healthier one. If you are like most people you take care of your car. You have the oil changed, you replace the worn tires, you put in the right gas. Why? Because you want it to be reliable and not break down on you. You want it to last longer, you want it to run efficiently, to get you from one place to the next as easily as possible. Well, your body is the vehicle that is taking you through life, your whole life. Surely you want it to be reliable, not to break down on you. You certainly want it to last longer, because there's no trading it in. You want it to run efficiently, getting you through life as easily as possible.

So, treat your body with the love and respect that it deserves. Think of it as your faithful servant. It is always there. When you get out of bed in the morning you put your feet on the floor and they support you. They may ache or hurt a little from the excess weight they are having to bear, but they do their best. And so it is with all your organs. They do the best they can with what they are given to work with. Give them the best you can and they will respond gratefully.

"Our bodies communicate to us clearly and specifically, if we are willing to listen to them."

———

SHAKTI GAWAIN

C IS FOR CONTROL

This is not the kind of control where you want to take over someone else's life. I'm talking about having control of what you can control and, generally speaking, that's yourself and your eating habits. Usually, you control what you eat and how much you eat. No one wants to be controlled by another person so why allow yourself to be controlled by a substance? When you take back control you let go of any blame that you have put on others for things that have happened to you. When you take control, you have the power to change. You *can* take control; you *can* make the changes needed to achieve your goal.

I have a colleague whose sister is in assisted living and cannot exercise. She is overweight. She cannot control *what* she eats because her meals are put in front of her so she exercises the only control she has... *how much* she eats. She has released 8 pounds in two months.

So, take control and focus on the empowerment that you feel. It's heady stuff! So many people who have control of the other factors in their life allow themselves to be controlled by their eating habits, but you *can* take control.

C IS FOR CHOICE

You are now going to make choices about the food you eat. Each and every day you make choices about who you are, every decision you make is one in which you decide who you are.

When I go to a department store and walk around holding a lipstick in my hand, I know that I could easily slip it into my large purse. However, I go to the checkout and pay for the lipstick because I am deciding that I am an honest person.

Every time you make a choice about what you eat you are deciding who you are. Who are you? Are you the overweight person, uncomfortable in their own skin, or the person who is in control and chooses to be slender and healthier?

I choose to have
a healthy slim body

C IS FOR COMMITMENT

Yes, getting yourself on the right road to reach your goal will require commitment; commitment to a new attitude towards food and eating. So what commitment are you really making when you decide to eat a small handful of nuts instead of that layer cake covered in cream? You are making a commitment to yourself, to give yourself the best opportunity to have a healthy body, to have freedom and flexibility of movement. You are making a commitment to feeling better about how you see yourself. You are making a commitment to experiencing more pleasure when you look in the mirror. You are making a commitment to you!

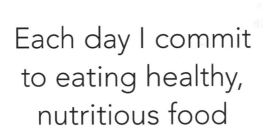

Each day I commit
to eating healthy,
nutritious food

D IS FOR DESIRE

There is a law in physics, the law of dominant effect. The desire that is greater is the desire that will overpower the weaker desire. Your desire to be slim, trim and healthy must be strong.

According to Dr. Judith Beck of the Beck Institute for Cognitive Behavior Therapy, and author of The Beck Diet Solution, you have two psychological muscles; the resistance muscle and the give-in muscle. When you make a decision to eat or not eat a certain food you are flexing one of these two muscles. The more you use the resistance muscle, for example, the stronger it becomes and the give-in muscle then becomes weaker through non-use. Flex that resistance muscle. Let your desire to be healthy and slim overcome any desire to eat in an inappropriate way!

"Desire is the starting point of all achievement, not a hope, not a wish but a keen pulsating desire which transcends everything."

___

NAPOLEON HILL

D IS FOR DEPRIVATION

Nobody likes to feel deprived, especially when it comes to food. And there is no need to feel deprived. When you are getting rid of all those extra pounds you are taking control of your life and your eating habits. You are gaining health, confidence, and freedom. Eating less is a positive!

If you are making a lifestyle change, it must be one that can be sustained. If you feel deprived you will very likely feel resentful and have that cookie, or extra serving, saying to yourself "Why shouldn't I have it? Who's to say I can't have it?" If you find yourself reaching for a snack, take a moment to say to yourself "Stop. I can take it or leave it. I will wait 15 – 20 minutes. If I still really want it then I can have it."

It is a fact that many times when we think we are experiencing hunger pangs we are actually thirsty and our body is dehydrated. So have a glass of water or another beverage and then re-examine if you still need to have that snack. If you do, eat something healthy and tasty, and if not stop thinking about food. Eat in moderation and never, ever allow yourself the feeling of deprivation.

D IS FOR DON'T EAT TO COMPLETE

Most of us have heard the phrase "You must finish everything on your plate… there are starving children in Africa/China." You feel that is the reason you are always compelled to clean your plate even though you are totally full and satisfied. However, there could be another reason why you feel you have to clean every last morsel on your plate. We have always been told to finish a task. As a child, if you were doing homework you were expected to complete it before going on to something else. When you make your bed, you don't make half of it and then decide not to finish it, do you?

We have an innate desire to complete a task we start and when we sit down to eat that is a task. When we open a bag of chips it feels uncomfortable to leave it half finished. How many times have you put the chip bag away half full only to feel that those chips are "'calling" you until you go in and finish them. Recognize your tendency to do this and either buy small packets of the things you eat or, if you buy in quantity, spend a few minutes re-packaging them into small packets. Then when you open one you will eat to complete and you will be done.

If, like many, you feel that it is more economical to buy in bulk, realize that it is more expensive to eat a whole bar of chocolate that costs $1.75 than a small wrapped piece of chocolate that costs 37 cents. Take a moment and check to see if you eat to complete.

E IS FOR ENJOYMENT

Enjoy the journey, enjoy the food you eat. Food metabolizes more efficiently when we are relaxed and stress-free. Nature intended that we eat, and we will be doing it all our lives, so eat food that you enjoy.

I had a client, whose diet consisted of hamburgers and French fries, who frowned and shook her head when it was suggested that she eat healthily. However, the fact is that just because you are making healthy choices you do not have to eat foods you dislike. You can find plenty of lists of healthy food on the internet.

Tufts University Health and Nutrition issued a list of 51 healthy foods you can say "yes" to and there are, of course, many more. Make your own list of foods that you enjoy and then check off those that support your healthy way of eating and living. You may be surprised at how many healthy choices you really enjoy!

E IS FOR EVERY DAY

Every day is a new day, a new opportunity. Yesterday has come and gone. Whatever you did then, or thought then, was then. Let it be. There is no need to repeat any of the ways that did not bring you the result you desired, and that includes your thoughts. Let your thoughts be positive.

Today is a new day. An opportunity to choose differently. As a client of mine put it so beautifully, "The sun comes up on a brand-new day every 24 hours, incredible huh?" How fortunate we are to have a new day every 24 hours, another chance to make new choices.

I see every day as a
new opportunity
to make new choices

E IS FOR EXERCISE

You are told over and over again that you have to exercise. If you want to shed weight, you hear that you must exercise regularly and consistently. So, when a client tells me that their goal is to exercise 6 or 7 days a week for 1 – 2 hours, I ask if they think it is sustainable *for the rest of their life.*

When one is carrying a lot of extra pounds around it is not easy to walk a mile. It can be tiring to walk around the block! So, what happens when you set an unrealistic goal and then find you can't keep it? You feel that you have failed. Do not set yourself up for that feeling. Make your exercise goal 3 minutes. Yes that's 3 *minutes* two or three times a week. You know you can do that easily, but you will find that you don't always stop at 3 minutes. You go a little longer – and feel you have succeeded. So, the next thing you know, you are doing 10 minutes and if one day you don't feel like doing 10 minutes and go back to even just 3 minutes you will still feel good because you have still reached your goal.

So be kind to yourself. Set realistic goals for exercising, and probably the most important thing you can do is see exercise as fun. Find something that you just love to do. Very often it is a sport, or something that you can do with a partner. Maybe you will join a dance class, go swimming or take a yoga class. Yoga is wonderful for the mind and marvelous for the body. Then there is always the best exercise of all, walking. Consider getting a Fitbit or Apple Watch to track your progress. Up to 5,000 steps a day is considered sedentary, 7,000 – 10,000 steps a day is moderate exercise. Studies have shown that measuring your steps greatly increases the amount of walking a person does, but once again do not set yourself goals that turn it into a stress. Take it easy if you want, and perhaps on a certain day you will choose to walk a little faster, go a little further. Remember that you are not in training for a marathon – or maybe you will be one of these days!

E IS FOR EXCUSES

If you are serious about letting go of your excess weight, if you are *really* serious about it, stop making excuses. I hear them all and the most common is "Well, I've been stressed." Well, guess what, aren't we all stressed in some form or another? Life is a process of change and any change is stressful, even good change. A renowned motivational speaker was approached by someone asking how they could be without stress, with no challenges at all. He replied that he could show them a place where they could be totally stress-free. The person was delighted until the gentleman said he would take them to the cemetery. "You will have no stress once you are there," he told them. Even people who appear to be totally carefree and seem to have everything possible to be stress free, have some stress in their lives. You can learn to handle stress without eating.

How often do you say "I don't have time to plan my meals. I don't have time to exercise"? It is true that with the pressures of our lives today time is a precious commodity. But, do you have time to watch your favorite TV show? Do you have time to play computer games? Do you have time to spend in chat rooms? You can decide how you want to allocate your time. Indeed, it can be time saving to plan your meals for the week. You decide whether you really cannot afford the extra fifteen to twenty minutes that it takes to buy fresh fruit and vegetables. You can buy them pre-cut, pre-washed and all ready to cook now! How convenient is that!

Do you find yourself saying "Well, it runs in my family. My mother has diabetes, our family is prone to heart disease"? Yes, there is some truth to the idea that certain traits or characteristics are genetic. But, are you using this as an excuse not to take care of yourself? If so, why?

My mother became ill at age 50. She was overweight, she developed diabetes, a brain tumor, dementia – the list goes on and on. She passed away at age 66 of cancer and in her last 16 years had no quality of life. My father passed away at age 68 from cancer. When I approached those years, I was asked "With both your parents dying comparatively young aren't you concerned about your health and chances of longevity?" My reply was "Well there are times when genetics come into play, but the way I see it, I am me, and I am doing what I can to stay healthy in both body and mind. I am not my parents. I am living **my** life." Fortunately, I have outlived both my parents and I am in very good health, for which I am grateful. I value my health and freedom and I am thankful for it.

So, if there is a history of ill health in your family but you are still healthy as you read this book, do not become a fatalist and don't let family genetics become your excuse not to take care of yourself.

I have heard it said that excuses are well-planned lies. Think about it, and stop making excuses!

E IS FOR ENERGY

What is the first thought that comes to mind when you think of the word energy? For some it will be electrical power, for some it will be the amount of "get-up-and-go" we have. For others it will be about the energy that surrounds us, that attracts certain things into our lives. We all generate energy and like attracts like. So, what you focus on will attract that to you.

Do not focus on what you do not want. When you look in the mirror, don't say to yourself, "Oh I hate those thighs. Oh, I don't want to be this big." As you look at yourself focus on what you do want.

"I will love being a size 10. I am really going to like being able to go on long walks, play tennis, travel with ease and comfort, run after the grandchildren." Focus on whatever being slim and healthy is going to give you; all the positive aspects of your life and the freedom you will have.

I am energized
and focused
on my goal to be
slim and fit

E IS FOR EMOTIONAL EATING

Are you an emotional eater? Chances are you are nodding your head. And you are not alone. Of the clients I see, a good 90% have emotional eating as their number one trigger. It is so easy to label oneself an emotional eater – and then eat. We are all emotional at times. There is a saying "Love is the answer, whatever the question." I like to say that food is *not* the answer whatever the problem, except hunger.

When you think about it, whatever is causing you distress will not be cured by eating. You will have a temporary distraction and the problem will still be there, unless you are hungry. If you are hungry, eating satisfies the hunger, over-eating does nothing for your hunger or distress.

If you are sad, eating does not change the cause of your sadness. It may give a sense of temporary relief for a very short while, but my guess is that after you have eaten that box of cookies, you are still sad.

If you are anxious, eating will not cause the anxiety to go away. So, look for ways to deal with your emotions without resorting to food. It is possible, you know.

F IS FOR FUN

So, do you like to have fun? "Of course'" you say. Then why continue to live in a way that could cause you to lose the ability to have fun as you age? Does that really make sense? Do you want to become a prisoner in your own body? Of course not. Then why continue to live in a way that may cause you to become just that?

Look for ways to have fun, small ways to enjoy a little levity. Find humor in everyday situations and have fun. Where is it written that striding down the road to health and freedom cannot be fun? It will be what you choose to make it.

"Never ever underestimate the importance of having fun."

———

RANDY PAUSCH

F IS FOR FIBER

Do you have enough fiber in your diet? If you are an average American the answer will be no. Our ancestors ate an astonishing 100 grams of fiber daily, which they obtained from their diet of fruit, nuts, fresh vegetables and a little very lean meat and fish. Now the average American has a mere 14 grams or so per day. The American Dietetic Association recommends at least 20 – 35 grams a day for healthy adults.

High-fiber foods tend to contain more nutrients and fewer calories. They are digested more slowly, and help us feel full sooner and recent research suggests that fiber can actually flush calories out of the body before they end up on the stomach or hips.

So, fill up on fiber and notice the effect!

F IS FOR FUEL

Food is fuel for your body, nothing more, nothing less. That is all nature has ever intended it to be. We have made it into so many things it was never intended to be; a comforter when we are sad, a reward when we have achieved something, a pacifier when we are hurt, a distraction when we are bored. But food does not solve any problem we experience, other than hunger. If you are bored and eat something, you may be distracted for a minute or two but then you are bored again.

Food is fuel for the body, so let's look once again to the analogy of your body being likened to your motor vehicle. Most people take very good care of their motor vehicles. They put in the right fuel, after all you would not put diesel into a gas car, would you? What would happen if you did? The car would be sluggish, it would not run properly. That is what happens when we put the wrong food (fuel) into our bodies. And do you go to a gas station, fill up with gas, drive down to the next corner, see another gas station and just **have** to try to squeeze more gas into your car? No, of course not. It doesn't make sense.

Why does it make sense then to fill your body, hopefully with the right fuel, and then, just because it is there, overfill it, stuff it full, squeeze in just a little more? Your body needs the right fuel, in the right amount, at the right time. It's that simple.

F IS FOR FEAR

Fear of failure. We all prefer not to fail. So many people who have been on diets feel they have failed. They lost weight, sometimes many pounds, only to gain it back when they went off the diet. Now they are afraid they are going to fail again. I ask you to think about what you are going to do right now in a different way. Just because you had a negative experience with long term results from dieting doesn't mean it will happen now. Now you are a different person to the one who went on the diet. We all change, constantly. We are not the same person we were a year ago, a month ago, a week ago. What you did then was try something that didn't work for you – then.

Edison and his team of scientists tried hundreds of filaments for the light bulb but each one didn't last long enough; it only gave a second or two of light. When they finally found a way to make a long-lasting light bulb, he was asked how he felt to have finally succeeded after all the failures. He replied that he didn't feel he had failed all those past times, he was just finding out what didn't work, which was taking him that much closer to what would work. Perhaps that's how it is with you. Perhaps the circumstances in your life are different now. Perhaps your motivation has increased. Perhaps you are just ready finally to be slender and healthy.

"There is only
one thing that
makes a dream
impossible to achieve;
the fear of failure."

**PAULO COELHO,
THE ALCHEMIST**

G IS FOR GAINING FREEDOM

Weight loss in itself is just that, weight loss. What you are looking for is what the end result does for you, what it gives you – quality of life.

What does quality of life give you? Quality of life brings freedom of movement. Everyday chores become easier. You are able to do seemingly small things like putting on your shoes with more ease, walk a little further without being out of breath, travel more comfortably. Think of all the ways carrying that extra weight restricts you from doing things you would like to do, or makes it harder to do those things that you have to do. Quality of life gives you freedom from the constant obsessive thoughts of food, from the feeling of being out of control, from feeling powerless.

Think about the freedom you will gain as you get rid of the excess pounds. Anticipate the sheer pleasure of feeling free to move easily.

G IS FOR GIFT

We all love to get gifts. A gift makes us feel special, loved and cared for. What is one of the best gifts you can give to those around you? Think about it. Yes, that's it. YOUR good health. When you are healthy it relieves those who care about you of the worry and anxiety they feel when you are sick or incapacitated. So, when you take care of yourself the gift to your family is freedom from concern.

In this day and age each family has so much to think about and be concerned about. Of course, eating and being slim is no guarantee that at some time you won't have physical challenges. However, by taking care of yourself, by doing the best you can to have a healthy body, you are giving those you love freedom from worry and concern. What a **wonderful** gift to our family and friends!

H IS FOR HEALTH

How great it is! In a recent survey of senior citizens, the number one thing that contributed to their quality of life was not wealth but health. You can have all the money in the world sitting in the bank, but if you are sitting in bed unable to breathe or move freely, your quality of life is impaired. I think of the story of a wealthy actress. She was beautiful and revered and left many, many millions in her estate and yet her last 10 years or so were spent in a wheelchair. She was a prisoner in her body and all her money could not free her.

What do you want to be thinking about when you go on vacation? "Do I have my sun lotion? Did I pack my new sandals?" Or "How many syringes will I need for my insulin? Do I have enough pills if we are delayed somewhere? I must be sure to know where the nearest emergency clinic is in case I need it."

Health is:

- Getting up from the chair easily and effortlessly.
- Taking a stroll in the evening summer sun without pain and discomfort.
- Breathing in cool mountain air freely.
- Laughing with the sheer joy of being alive and well.
- Swimming with dolphins on your 70th birthday.
- Dancing to whatever music touches your soul.
- Playing a spot-on game of golf.

The list goes on and I know you can add many more of your own personal pleasures. Isn't being able to do any of those things worth more to you than one extra helping, one piece of sugar-laden cake, or a large French fries, rather than a small one? Remember – nothing tastes as good as slim and healthy feels!

H IS FOR HONESTY

Be honest with yourself. Why are you holding on to that excess fat? Everyone says "I don't want to be overweight." So why are you? Could it be that you are subconsciously not wanting to outshine someone around you, a spouse, a sister, mother, daughter, brother? I was told by a client "Well, I've thought in the past that if I succeed in shedding weight my daughter will feel badly because she isn't able to." I asked this woman how her daughter was doing now and she said her daughter had let go of some weight. I asked "So if your daughter was overweight at the moment would you be here?" She smiled sheepishly and said "Probably not."

If you feel this way you may take some steps towards healthy eating, but you will probably sabotage yourself. But you have a right to be slender and healthy. You are doing yourself and that other person a disservice by not giving yourself the best chance, the best honest chance to let go of unhealthy fat and be the slim person you want to be, have a right to be. You could well find that by setting an example, by shining your light so to speak, those around you will benefit from being in that light and begin to shine more themselves.

So be honest with yourself. Look at your motivations and possible blockages that are stopping you from reaching your goal.

H IS FOR HUNGER

Are you afraid of being hungry? If so, you are not alone. We have come to fear being hungry. It amazes me how many commercials I hear or read about for weight loss and one of the overriding perks is that "you will never feel hungry again." You can swill down the shakes and lose the weight, until you stop taking the shakes of course. Then you will want and need to get back into eating regular food, for you cannot sustain yourself indefinitely on shakes, and the weight will pile back on. You won't have achieved your goal of a permanently healthy, slim you but you will never be hungry! So why do we see hunger as a negative, when in fact it is just a signal from nature that we need to re-fuel. It is sometimes said that hunger is the physical need for food, while appetite is the psychological desire for food. Hunger is of the body; appetite is of the mind. Feed the hunger of the body.

Are you saying to yourself "But I can't tell when I am truly hungry and I also have a problem with knowing when I am full and satisfied"? Certain physical sensations can trigger eating behavior. Your stomach may growl, or you may feel stomach contractions, for example. Learn to be in tune with your body. Listen to it.

When you eat, part of the food is converted to glucose, and your blood sugar level rises rapidly. This prompts the release of insulin, a hormone that helps move circulating blood sugar into fat storage. Insulin filters slowly into the spinal fluid and when it reaches a certain level, a "full" signal is sent to the brain. For most people it takes about 20 minutes from the beginning of eating for feelings of fullness to begin. From this you will see that eating more slowly helps the stomach to signal to the brain that it is full. Learning to distinguish when you are actually hungry and when you are actually fully satisfied can help you to control your eating portions.

H IS FOR HYPNOSIS

There are many myths regarding hypnosis, many of them perpetuated by Hollywood movies. Having been a Certified Hypnotherapist for many years, let me assure you that hypnosis is totally safe and you are **never** under the control of the hypnotist. With hypnosis, which is a very deep state of relaxation, a trained hypnotherapist accesses the subconscious mind which gives you help in making choices that will take you in the direction you want to go, be it weight control, fear of driving, anxiety or many other issues. Suggestions are made to change some of those long-standing habits, and re-frame some of the beliefs you have about yourself and your ability to let go of your excess weight and your eating habits.

Like any weight-loss program, hypnosis is not a silver bullet but it has been proven to be highly successful in assisting those who truly want to be slender and healthy. If you decide on this route, find a hypnotherapist you are comfortable with who offers the program that will work for you. In my practice I offer two weight loss programs: One for people who want to let go of an irksome few extra pounds and the Gastric *Mind* Band program, an amazing and revolutionary program from Europe for those who have a substantial amount of weight to release. So, look around and find the hypnotherapist that you would like to work with and check out hypnosis. See if it feels right for you. It works!

I IS FOR IMAGINATION

The subconscious mind does not differentiate between reality and something vividly imagined. So, when your mind imagines something over and over again it begins to believe that it has actually happened.

It is said that imagination is the language of the subconscious mind. The more you imagine the end result the more likely you are to bring it about.

Some people can imagine in breathtakingly vibrant colors. Others imagine in black and white. Some people cannot "see" it at all. If that is you, *feel* the results of being slim. Feel how it would be to walk easily, effortlessly and quickly. Feel how it would be to reach down to pick a flower or pick up a ball. Imagine how it will feel to be lithe and energetic. Imagine and feel, if you can, how great it will be to be able to perform easily and effortlessly the tasks that now take up much of your time and effort.

I IS FOR INVEST IN YOURSELF

I have had clients who have said "You know, it's expensive to eat healthily." And my answer to that is "You know, it's also expensive to be sick."

A survey showed that $20 went a lot further on healthy food than it did on fast food. Fast food – or fake food, as we should think of it – is not inexpensive in the long run, especially when one considers the effect it can have on health. Yes, it is convenient most of the time. However, with just a little planning, a little foresight, you can put together lunches or snacks for less than you will pay going through a fast food drive up. Use the crock-pot so that meals are waiting for you when you get home after you've had a long and busy day. Spend a little extra time planning healthy and tasty meals for yourself and see the benefits.

Invest in yourself. Take care of yourself. You're worth it.

I IS FOR ICE CREAM

"What?" you say. "What are you talking about? How can I have ice cream when I want to lose weight?" Well, here we go back to the basic premise that you are not going to be deprived. You will make choices and if you choose to eat ice cream today, tomorrow you can make a different choice. You may read labels and choose an ice cream that is natural and has less sugar. All ice cream is not created equal.

You will also decide how much ice cream you are going to eat. Do you **really** need to eat a whole tub of ice cream? Can you **really** be that hungry? Probably not, so have a small portion if you have decided that is what you really want. Just remind yourself that you will make a different choice tomorrow.

I am in control
of what I eat
and how much I eat

I IS FOR "I AM"

Research suggests that approximately 70% of our thoughts are negative. Now the mind cannot have two thoughts at the same time. It cannot sustain a negative and positive thought at the same time. This powerful exercise was given to me by a friend, Cristine Hueyke.

If I begin to doubt myself and things happening in my life, I go through this exercise:

Begin each sentence with I AM. Go through the letters of the alphabet finding a positive adjective for every letter. The words can be said out loud, or silently to yourself. It doesn't matter if you believe what you are saying. It is not about convincing yourself that you are all the positive things you think of. If you feel you have to "buy into" what you are saying you may start to analyze and even refute it, making it non-effective. So, treat it as a word game. A positive word game!

For example:

I am... Attractive... Awesome... Agile...
I am... Brave... Beautiful... Benevolent...
I am... Clever... Cheerful... Charismatic...
And so on...

You may want to only find one adjective for each letter each time you do the exercise or you may want to find as many as possible.

If a negative word comes to mind, as it may, just erase it and find a positive word. It becomes so interesting as you come up with a new word every now and again that you may wonder "Where did that come from?" Try it, it's fun and it's good for you!

J IS FOR JUST DO IT

Stop procrastinating. Make it happen. The journey of a thousand miles begins with one step, so take that first step. Yes, there is always tomorrow, but why not start right now. Think about being on a journey. You are starting on a journey, a journey to health and freedom. Take the first step. You don't have to change everything overnight.

Consider the fable of the tortoise and the hare. Tortoise and Hare decided to have a race. Hare strutted around laughing at Tortoise. "How can you possibly think you can beat me?" he asked Tortoise. "You are so slow you don't have a chance." Hare raced off, leaving Tortoise to plod along in his own slow way. When Hare was far ahead, he felt tired and decided he had time to take a quick nap. That quick nap turned into a deep sleep and as he lay sleeping Tortoise plodded by and reached the winning post first.

Just do it, just take the first step.

"Life is not a spectator sport. If watching is all you're gonna do, then you're gonna watch your life go by without you."

FROM THE HUNCHBACK OF NOTRE DAME

J IS FOR JOY

You have a right to your joy! Does being overweight bring you joy?

Helen Keller once said "Life is either a wonderful adventure or it is nothing."

Why would you not have a wonderful adventure? You can never get anywhere if you are not prepared to take that first step. This is not about climbing Mount Everest. This is about taking control of your eating habits. So, if being overweight brings you no joy, take off on your adventure into good health, vitality, fulfillment and joy.

Feel the joy of being slender, healthy and free! Go for it – you are worth it!

I choose to be joyful
right here, right now

K IS FOR KEEP GOING

Do you sometimes feel that you are a quitter? Have you tried something and then just given up? Very likely. Most of us have. If you take just one thing with you from reading this book, make it that this is a journey for life. In my experience, there is no quick fix that is long-lasting when it comes to shedding weight. So, make up your mind right at the beginning that you are going to keep going and not quit. The only person who fails to get rid of their excess weight is the person who gives up.

Perhaps you have heard about the family who left Albuquerque during the Depression and traveled day by day across New Mexico and Arizona in the blazing sun with the intention of reaching the ocean, San Diego to be exact. Each day they thought they must surely be there and each day they were not. Finally, they decided they had made a mistake and were not going to reach San Diego so they turned around and went back to Albuquerque. Little did they know that they were approaching El Centro, that they were a mere 200 miles from their destination. So, having traveled nearly 1,000 miles they turned back and traveled another 1,000 miles just to be back where they started. So close! So, keep on keeping on – keep going.

K IS FOR KNOWLEDGE

The idea of knowledge is not that one should immerse oneself in all the fine details of nutrition and wellness necessarily. You can let the experts do that, but knowing certain basic information about eating in a healthy way is so beneficial and can even be fun.

Do you know, for example, that 4.2 grams of sugar is the equivalent of one teaspoon of sugar? Most of my clients are not aware of that so when reading a label and seeing 20 grams of sugar they do not equate that to almost 5 teaspoons of sugar. It sounds a lot more when put that way, doesn't it? Do you know that approximately 13 almonds are 75 calories? Now, although the idea is not to count calories and I do not recommend that to my clients, it can be useful to have that knowledge at the back of your mind as you reach for a handful of almonds for your snack.

"Knowledge is Power" as the saying goes, and you are in the process of taking back your power; your power to make wise and beneficial choices to support you in reaching your goal.

I go through each
day choosing
healthy, nutritious food

L IS FOR LAUGHTER

How's your Laugh Life? Okay, in the past you may have felt that you "slipped up", you had a lapse. In your new way of looking at life, try laughing at yourself. It is not the end of the world, don't take yourself too seriously! Remember, all you have done is made a choice. You may think it wasn't the best one but see if you can laugh at yourself, laugh at the situation.

Look for the humor, the irony and absurdity of life in a tough, stressful situation. This will help improve your mood and the mood of those around you. Where is it said that life has to be dreary, that we have to stress over so many things? Certainly, there are situations that are just plain sad, difficult and tense. Food didn't improve those times so try a little old-fashioned laugh at life! They say that laughter is the best medicine, so look for the positive. If things get tough, and they usually do for most of us at some time, forget about turning to food, it's not the answer. See if there is anything, any small thing that can cause you to laugh or at the very least, smile.

Studies have shown that just 15 minutes of laughter a day will burn 10 to 40 calories, depending on a person's weight and the intensity of the laughter. That's enough to shift between 1 and 4 pounds a year. Obviously, you're not burning thousands of calories, but as anyone who has let go of that unwanted weight knows, it's little changes that make a big difference. Plus, having a laugh usually makes a person feel more positive about life – and ultimately, this can help you to feel better about yourself and make you more motivated to release those excess pounds. So – lighten up and laugh!

L IS FOR LOVE

Love your body, love yourself, love your food, love your life! Yes, you may want to weigh a whole lot less than you do at this moment. You may look in the mirror and feel unhappy with what you see there, but your body is doing the best it can with what it is given, so love your body, just know it will be a more slender, fitter, stronger body down the road.

- Find time to love yourself. It is not only okay to love yourself, it's desirable that you love yourself. It's not grandiose or boastful or unseemly. When you love yourself you take better care of yourself. Don't you always try to take really good care of something, or someone, that you love? Make yourself one of those people that you love!
- Love your food. We were meant to enjoy our food; it is the means of our survival. When you have mastered the art of moderation you will be able to love your food without the need to over-indulge.
- Love your life. Life is short and you can choose how you see it. We all have challenges but we influence our reality by the thoughts we choose to have about it. So, love your life for the miracle that it is. It is the only one you have!

"We love life, not
because we are
used to living,
but because we are
used to loving."

———

FRIEDRICH NIETZSCHE

M IS FOR **METABOLISM**

Your Resting Metabolic Rate is the amount of calories needed just to keep your body functioning. Any calories above that will increase your weight. Find ways to supercharge your metabolism.

- Drink plenty of water. A consistent intake of 6 – 8 glasses a day will enhance your metabolism to the tune of about an extra 100 calories a day – about 11 pounds a year! An easy and efficient way to let go of those pounds.
- Exercise after you eat. Exercise done about an hour after a meal can actually be more beneficial than if it is done before the meal. During a phenomenon called "Dietary Induced Thermogen" the body burns about 50% more calories on a full stomach than it does on an empty one.
- Avoid high-refined carbohydrate intake. There are two kinds of carbohydrates: "complex" such as fresh vegetables, fruits and nuts and "simple" or refined" such as white bread, pasta, rice, cookies, refined sugars, and crackers. We need carbohydrates in our diet but trying to let go of weight on a low-fat, high-carbohydrate diet often does not work. A diet of complex carbohydrates along with protein from fish and some lean meat will inhibit the rapid release of insulin and facilitate the burning of fat.
- Try a whiff of strawberries. It has been found that this increases your metabolism! The Smell and Taste Treatment Research Foundation in Chicago states that if you take a stroll surrounded by the scent of strawberries it can boost your metabolism by 20%. Strange but true, they say.

M IS FOR MOTIVATION

What is your motivation? There are two kinds of motivation – the carrot and the stick. The carrot is the something positive that you are going to attain – freedom of movement as you become more slender, the ease with which you can perform daily tasks, relief of pain as your joints are not overburdened, the feeling of pleasure and wellness as you look in the mirror and see the person you want to be, the person you are choosing to be.

The stick is the motivation of what can happen to you if you continue to eat obsessively and remain overweight. Some of the illnesses associated with obesity are diabetes, stroke, heart disease, sleep apnea and now research is indicating that people with diabetes may have a higher risk of Alzheimer's. You may tell yourself you can deal with the physical disabilities that come from being obese but do you really want to risk losing your mind in order to have that extra donut, or that extra portion that you know you do not need?

Discover what **really** motivates you!

"Only I can change my life. No one can do it for me."

CAROL BURNETT

M IS FOR MEDITERRANEAN LIFESTYLE

It has been recorded that people in the Mediterranean region live longer, healthier lives than others. This is based on their eating habits. Most of their food is plant-based and includes the use of olive oil.

Here are a few suggestions that you may want to incorporate into your lifestyle:

- Eat a variety of unprocessed, home-cooked foods.
- Eat plant-based foods such as fruit, vegetables, whole grains, beans, lentils, nuts and seeds.
- It is recommended that you replace other fats, such as butter and margarine, with olive oil.
- Limit or avoid foods high in trans-fats (these foods will have the words "hydrogenated" or "partially-hydrogenated oils"). You will likely see them on the labels of crackers, cookies, cakes, pies and pastries.
- Eat two fish meals per week.
- Replace red meat with fish or poultry. Limit red meat to once or twice a week.
- Eat small amounts of dairy products daily. Be aware that cheese is very high in fat content.
- Eat fewer egg yolks. Use egg replacer or egg whites, with only an occasional egg yolk.

Please note that fast foods and convenience foods are not a part of the Mediterranean lifestyle!

And always consult your doctor or nutritionist before making a dietary change, especially if you are on medication.

M IS FOR MINDFUL EATING

Become mindful and take time to enjoy your food. Being mindful has many benefits. Being mindful keeps us in the present moment. Being mindful means that you are aware of what you are eating. So be in the moment when you are eating. Eat slowly, savoring every bite. We appear to have lost the art of mindful eating, as we rush from one event to another, from one task to another.

Take time to eat. Even if you are eating alone, consider setting the table with your best napkin, maybe a candle and your good silverware. Yes, you may find yourself reading a book as you eat, or even watching the television – neither of which is recommended – but setting the place at the table will help you to appreciate the meal you are about to enjoy.

I take time to
eat my food
slowly and mindfully

M IS FOR MOVEMENT

So often we have a resistance to the word "exercise", but exercise is just movement of the body. So now consider the amount of movement you do each day. The word exercise conjures up visions of hard work, sweating bodies and long lengths of time. Indeed, that kind of exercise can be very beneficial as you get the heart rate up.

However, taking life one day at a time, consider doing more body movement than you are at present. One very effective way is to play music, any kind of music that speaks to you and dance... yes, dance... to it... all by yourself. With no-one watching you are free to express yourself in any way you choose, so feel the music and swirl and twirl or just sway and play. Feel the rhythm and let your body move. Cover up the mirror; you don't need to watch yourself. You may feel like a top ballerina, or a cool hip-hop mover. Let your imagination take you wherever it will as you immerse yourself in the music that enchants you, and move to its beat!

If you are going to watch a TV show, instead of sitting down immediately, stand in front of the TV and raise your toes and heels, or do shoulder rolls for a few minutes **then** sit down. Keep it short and manageable, but move.

M IS FOR MAINTENANCE

It is easy once you have reached your goal to wonder what to do next. If your motivation was *only* to reach your goal weight, and not to change your way of thinking and way of life, you may find yourself unable to maintain your new healthy weight.

One thing you can do is anticipate being at your goal weight. Start new thin activities before you've let go of all the weight you want to shed. Play tennis, wear shorts, have a round or two of golf, get into yoga. People often think that if they become slim their lives will magically change, they will find a romantic partner, they will get a better job, they will have a better social life. While it is possible that these things can and will happen, it is possible that letting go of your weight may solve some problems but there will be others.

Do not put all your expectations into reaching your goal. It is just another road stop on your journey of life. Life will be more than just being slim. When you are getting close to your goal consider finding another goal that you can move towards, something that does not involve food. Then when you attain your goal weight you will continue to feel motivated by your new project. You may decide to tackle another aspect of your life that you have neglected through the many years of obsessing over food. You may decide to nourish your mind.

Be prepared for the feeling of exhilaration as you reach your goal and then perhaps a sense of anti-climax – what next? You may have become used to people commenting on how well you are doing, how great you look and now they are used to seeing the new you and no longer comment. Do not let that deter you from continuing to eat in a way that supports the new slim, healthy you.

N IS FOR NOW

Do it NOW! How often do we live in the past, how often do we try to live in the future? Don't put off doing the things you want to do until you've shed your excess weight. Look for things that you can and want to do... NOW. Life is lived NOW... not yesterday... not tomorrow. Now is all that you have.

There is a beautiful Zen story. There was once a man who was being chased by a ferocious tiger across a field. At the edge of the field there was a cliff. In order to escape the jaws of the tiger, the man caught hold of a vine and swung himself over the edge of the cliff. He felt the vine beginning to give way as he glanced down and saw, to his dismay that another tiger was waiting on the ground below him! He knew that at any second he could fall to certain death. At that moment, he noticed a wild strawberry plant growing in a crevice on the cliff. In the center of the plant was the most beautiful big red strawberry. Clutching the vine with one hand, he plucked the strawberry with the other and put it in his mouth. "Ah," he said "Bliss." He never before realized how sweet a strawberry could taste. Now that is definitely living in the moment!

"You are not meant to serve time. Time is meant to serve you. Become the master of your now."

———

E'YEN A. GARDNER

N IS FOR NO

Say it... "No." Say it again... "No." How does that feel? Were you, like so many people, taught as a child to be "good"? To do the right thing? Think about the "terrible twos." That's when a small child learns the power of saying "No." Whatever the request, they say it with glee "No!" However, they soon learn that "No" doesn't usually get them what they want so "No" becomes a negative word. We start to use it less and less. We want to conform; we want to be liked so we say "Yes."

However, take the time to be supportive of yourself and learn to say "No" when this is in your best interests. Each time you say "No" to a dessert that you actually don't want, feel the empowerment. When you say "No, I'm not going to buy that bar of chocolate" or "No, I won't have that snack at this moment" it empowers you. It's okay to say "No." It's more than okay. At times it is incredibly good to say "No." So, if saying "No" feels uncomfortable for you, practice. You'll find you could enjoy saying "No."

N IS FOR NATURE'S CANDY

What is nature's candy? Why, fruit, of course! The next time you are thinking of reaching for candy, just insert the word *nature's* in front of it. Fruits such as apples, melons, and berries are excellent snacks. Bananas should be eaten early in the day as they take a long time to digest and they are high in sugar. I generally recommend that a woman eats half a banana at one time as that gives the potassium needed and cuts back on the sugar intake.

Eat fruit for dessert if you are in the habit of having dessert. If possible, wait a while before having the fruit after you have eaten. This is better for the digestive system. Remember that fruit does contain a lot of sugar, albeit natural sugar, so keep your portions modest.

N IS FOR NUTRITION MISSION

When you go on a diet, the first thing you think of is what you cannot have. So often you stop eating those things which are labeled "bad." Sometimes these foods are nutritious, many times they are not. Part of the goal is to give your body the fuel it needs to keep you running efficiently and for as long as possible. The way to do that is to give it the right fuel, food that is nutritious.

Highly processed foods have most, if not all, of the nutrition taken out of them. When flour is sent to the manufacturers of baked goods the essential vitamins are removed and then sold to vitamin companies. Often three or four are put back in and the product is labeled "niacin enriched" or "iron fortified." These are vitamins that were taken out in the first place! Avoid goods that are composed of refined ingredients.

Go on a Nutrition Mission – have fun, try one new recipe per month. Choose something that is healthy but not too complicated, not too much work. And enjoy it!

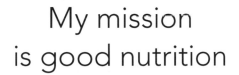

My mission
is good nutrition

O IS FOR OWN UP

Own up to yourself the things that are a challenge. Own up to the times you have dealt with challenges in a less than perfect way. You are not always going to make the right choices, that is what choice is about. However, it's not going to wreck your self-esteem to own up, so be honest with yourself. You could have made another choice, you didn't, but don't beat yourself up.

Most importantly, own up to yourself when you make excuses that allow you to eat inappropriately. Own up and then take responsibility for your actions. Once you own up to your actions you can move forward and make changes to produce the results you desire.

"Taking personal accountability is a beautiful thing because it gives us complete control of our destinies."

———

HEATHER SCHUCK, THE WORKING MOM MANIFESTO

O IS FOR OPPORTUNITY

We all have opportunities in life. Some we take advantage of and others we let pass us by. Every day you have an opportunity to take a different path, to make a change. How fortunate we are to have another day with fresh opportunities. This may be your very opportunity, right now, to change negative eating habits into positive eating habits. This may be your opportunity, right now, as Henry David Thoreau said, to go confidently in the direction of your dreams. If your dream is to be slim and healthy, go for it. You have the opportunity, right now!

"While we are making up our minds as to when we shall begin, the opportunity is lost."

—

QUINTILIAN

O IS FOR ONESELF

Do this for yourself; for you, not for anyone else. The saying goes "Nothing tastes as good as slim feels." How true!

I was in Paris once, 30 years or more ago, people watching, and saw a French woman stroll down the street. She was old, very old it seemed to me. Her face was as lined and wrinkled as a withered leaf, but she walked with head held high, holding the leash to her little dog, and it was apparent that she loved who she was. She was aware of herself as a woman. Inside she probably still felt she was 40 years old. I wondered at the time what made the difference between her and her English counterparts. They have the same weather, which involves rain and cold, but being raised in England I remembered that English women had a way of bundling up with a headscarf tied around their head, shopping bag in hand, trundling down the road. French women still seemed to be aware of their essence, whatever their age or size.

So be aware of who you are, extra weight and all! Celebrate your essence and don't apologize for who you are. Just resolve to be the slim person that you want to be and deserve to be. Do it for yourself for you **are** worth it.

I am already worthy
of that which I desire

P IS FOR PORTIONS

How big they are! A client lamented to me that she wondered why more women were overweight than men. Let us look at our national pastime of eating out. Americans love to eat out. Our portions are far larger than they were 20 years ago. Why? Because we are encouraged to overeat. When we eat in a restaurant, for example, we are served large plates of food. Why? Because we want perceived value. We want our money's worth.

All through life many women eat out with their partner, spouse, and friends. When the meal is ordered the chef in the kitchen receives an order for, let's say, two spaghettis. He serves two identical plates. It is not his job to wonder if they are for two men, one man and one woman, a woman and a youth. His job is to serve a plate that will satisfy the biggest hunger, that of the man usually. So, the woman will sit and eat mouthful for mouthful with the man. Is it any wonder that women are more overweight than men? The man is getting a portion more suitable to his size and weight, the woman is usually grossly overeating. The woman must decide how much food she is going to eat, the chef will not decide for her.

When eating meals at home serve the food in the kitchen and cover anything that is left. Never, ever eat directly out of a jar. If, for example, you love peanut butter, put a teaspoon or so into a bowl to eat. If you dip into the jar you could find half of it gone before you can say "knife."

Serve on a small plate. You eat less food when it is served on a small plate because the food itself automatically seems to be more. Try it! Also, psychologists have found that we eat less off a black plate, so try that small black plate and watch your portions – and your waistline – shrink!

P IS FOR PERSONAL POWER

How satisfying it is to feel that we have our own power: Personal Power. We do have it, you know. Only we can give that power away, either to someone else or to something else. Only we can take it back. Take back your Personal Power. When you are tempted to overeat or eat something that you feel is unhealthy, you can quietly say to yourself "Stop! Personal Power. I can take it or leave it. I think I will leave it." Or you may even decide to take it. That will be your choice, but you will have given yourself a chance to take back your Personal Power.

We had a severe storm recently and electricity was out for days. It was cold and bleak! The phrase most heard was "We've lost our power" but it was pointed out to me that the phrase should be "We have lost our electricity." We had not lost our power, our Personal Power. We still had it and we could choose how to utilize it. Utilize your Personal Power.

"Within you right now is the power to do things you never dreamed possible. This power becomes available to you just as soon as you can change your beliefs."

_____

MAXWELL MALTZ

P IS FOR POSTURE

There is a tendency for overweight people to hunch their shoulders forward and walk in a hesitant, almost apologetic way. Many overweight people feel judged. They unconsciously try to make themselves less noticeable. Next time you find a tendency to do this make a conscious effort to stand straight and tall, head up and shoulders back. This has some very positive benefits, one of which is that you will immediately seem slimmer. You will also *feel* slimmer and feel better about yourself. You have no reason to slouch and make yourself more diminished. No matter how much you weigh you are a very valuable human being and have a right to as much self-worth and respect as any slim person. Try it – it feels good!

As I stand tall
and straight,
I feel slimmer

P IS FOR PLATEAU

During the course of your weight reduction you will have one or more plateaus. This is a normal occurrence. Your body is adjusting to its new set point. The set point is the weight to which the body becomes accustomed, no matter how much you might disagree with it. A plateau usually lasts a week or two but for some it can last three to four weeks, or even longer. However, the metabolism will rise again, the plateau will pass and weight loss resumes. Here is a very important point to remember. When you reach your goal weight the body still remembers its set-point weight and seeks to regain it. It may take anywhere from six months to a year for the body to accept the goal weight as its new set point.

Patience and persistence are very important at this time and exercise is a very good way of shortening and overcoming the periodic plateaus that you will experience. If you have a reinforcement download, listen to it more often and then just relax and know that you are still on the journey. You have reached a resting spot. Take this opportunity to give yourself credit for what you have accomplished so far. Realize that perfection in all you do is not as important as living life one step at a time, one day at a time, and enjoying the new plateau. Give yourself permission to reward yourself with happy, positive and healthful thoughts as you rest at the plateau. Formulate and update realistic goals to guide you to the next step in your food plan and processes. Continue to think slim, slender, and healthy and just relax. The plateau will pass!

Q IS FOR QUICKLY

We are a society that expects instant gratification. Communication has become instant and we expect to see the results of our efforts quickly. However, weight loss seldom happens in that way. Yes, you can drop weight quickly with a diet, but the weight that is released slowly and steadily will stay off permanently because you will be forming healthy eating habits.

I tell my clients that hypnosis is not a quick fix. It is not a magic wand, but hypnosis helps you to re-form your ideas and beliefs about food and eating. On a conscious level you can reinforce your commitment to letting go of the weight by regularly re-affirming your willingness to go forward steadily, eating in a normal and natural way.

Remember that you are on a journey and it may take time, but you can and will reach your destination.

I am patient and
persistent.
I eat naturally and
normally on my
journey to a
slender body.

Q IS FOR QUALITY OF LIFE

What do you want in life? What constitutes quality of life for you? Is it really eating two tubs of ice cream or six donuts, and then looking in the mirror and disliking what you see? Is it really feeling frustrated as you watch the pounds pile onto your body? Is it really packing your holiday suitcase and making sure you have enough medications in case you are stranded somewhere and have to stay an extra day or two?

Is it quality of life to be wondering if you are going to be able to keep up with the rest of the group? I heard of a group of students who were having a tour of Washington State University. One member of the group was so overweight that she was unable to keep up with the group; she straggled behind and finally was totally lost. I imagine that was not a good feeling for her, not one she would have chosen.

It is not a sin to be overweight but it can certainly be inconvenient and frustrating. Is that what you consider quality of life? As I've said before, healthy eating and weight release do not guarantee that you will live totally free from any health challenges all your life. However, you will be giving yourself the very best chance of having a quality life and surely you deserve that?

Q IS FOR QUIET DETERMINATION

What kind of person are you? Do you decide to do something and broadcast it to the world? Do you decide and keep it to yourself, almost as a cherished secret? Whatever works for you is the way for you to go. However, there is strength in quiet determination. What is quiet determination? Firstly, it does not include "I wonder if I can" or "Perhaps I'll give it a try." Determination is resolve, solid resolve. It will be done. I can do it. I will do it. Quiet determination is the resolve that is decided within. It doesn't have to be proclaimed from the rooftops. There is a train of thought that says it is better to share your goals with others so that you are held accountable by your words. However, perhaps that puts too much pressure on you. Not everyone wants to be examined by their friends and family so that they feel they are living life under a microscope.

I have found that there is a delicious pleasure in secretly going forward towards a goal. When I do, the journey is mine, and I am not doing this for anyone but me. Certainly, I know my family are happy to see me slimmer and possibly healthier but this is my journey, my destination and I can answer to me. I don't need to answer to anyone else. So, see if this appeals to you. If it does, go forward in quiet determination; no bells, no fanfare, just you going forward knowing that you are on the road to your destination of health and freedom.

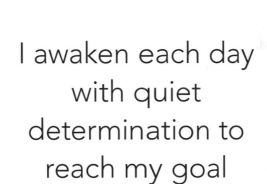

I awaken each day
with quiet
determination to
reach my goal

R IS FOR REGRET

If there is a sad word in the English language it has to be regret. Regret that you did or did not do something and later regret the decision.

Do you want to get towards the end of your life and regret...? that you abused your body... that you didn't respect yourself enough to take care of your physical body... that you overate, grew overweight?

How does this sound to you? *"I wish I didn't have Type 2 diabetes... I wish I could climb that step... I wish I wasn't in so much pain... I wish... I wish..."* Not great, is it? Well, it doesn't have to be like that. You can make the changes you need to make right now.

It's been said before "This is not a dress rehearsal." If you are lucky you will reach old age. As you age you may have health challenges, and I believe we are encouraged to think that aging automatically brings infirmity, but that is not necessarily so. There are many very elderly people who are in excellent health and leading a quality life. Why couldn't that be *you*? Why shouldn't that be *you*? Why wouldn't that be *you*?

Of course, there are no guarantees, but if you do lead a balanced, healthy life and at some time you have to deal with health challenges you will not also have the pain of regret. Make the decision right now to give yourself the best shot at a full life and eliminate regret.

R IS FOR REMEMBER

Remember who you are and who you really want to be, who you deserve to be. Perhaps you were not overweight as a child. Why have you allowed yourself to gain all this excess baggage? Think back to the joy of being slim and lithe. Remember the feeling of freedom you had as a child. Many of my clients say that they always thought they were chubby as a child but when they look back now, they realize that they weren't. Remember what it was like when you felt great, when you were in control of your habits. Remember and resolve to feel that way again. Why would you settle for less?

If you have never been slim, recall a time when you were extremely happy. Perhaps you were by yourself, playing in the sand and you were oblivious to your size. You were just you, a child, having a grand old time. If you can remember such a time, recreate that feeling, hold on to it and at the same time imagine yourself slim. Put aside the size you are now, hold on to that glorious feeling that you had when you were so happy, so enthralled with what you were doing that your size did not matter at all. Then in that instance imagine yourself as slender.

S IS FOR SUGAR

How sweet it is – NOT! Have you really looked at labels to see how much sugar you are actually consuming? In 1828 sugar intake amounted to an average of 7 lbs per person per year. In 2012 according to the U.S. Department of Agriculture, the average American's sugar intake was an incredible 160 lbs per year!

There is as much sugar in a single can of cola as in five pounds of venison which was a staple of our ancestors' diet and would have taken them a week or more to consume. There's more sugar in a super size side of fries than in five pounds of elk!

In nature, sugar content was closely proportional to the available fat and protein in each meal. The rise in free sugar, that is the starch in the bloodstream after a meal, is a remarkably accurate indicator of how many calories were just consumed. That's why it became the most important control signal for your digestion, not the only one, but the most important. Since there isn't much free sugar in nature, a small rise in sugar signals the end of a pretty big meal. But this carefully balanced response developed over hundreds of millions of years by fish and animals, including humans, goes crazy in a fast-food world. Before we invented agriculture, we ate over two hundred different plants, fruits and nuts and as many as a hundred different game animals, snakes, worms and insects. There was very little starch or sugar in any of them. Now everything we consume contains sugar.

So again, read labels. When something is low in fat it usually has a high sugar content. If you need to sweeten use a healthy sugar alternative whenever possible. If you do eat sugar, use raw sugar instead of refined sugar. The best solution is to gradually wean yourself off the taste of sweet substances, so that your taste buds are satisfied by foods that are not too sweet.

S IS FOR SALT

Most people will say that they do not eat too much salt. However, the amount of salt in the average American diet is about 3,400 milligrams, three quarters of which comes not from the salt shaker but from processed foods. The Federal Dietary Guidelines recommends 2,300 mg of salt per day and 1,500 mg for the elderly.

Our body does require salt, but too much sodium in our diet can lead to health problems. One of these is high blood pressure which leads to heart attacks and stroke, water retention and kidney stones.

What can one do to cut back on salt intake? One report suggests that bread is the culprit for many Americans. This is not necessarily because there is so much salt in it, just that we eat too much bread that has salt. Try to avoid processed foods and if you do buy them check the labels. Our palate becomes accustomed to heavily salted foods and it may seem difficult to cut out salt altogether, so look for salt substitutes that contain less sodium. There are many, but my favorite is Bragg Liquid Aminos, which has a quarter of the sodium of table salt. Sea salt is also an acceptable alternative. If you want to use salt, stay away from refined table salt. Use spices more liberally and you will find yourself using less salt. Read labels and become aware of how much salt you are actually consuming each day.

S IS FOR SLOW

Nice and easy does it... Yes, you want to be one of those people who are 90 lbs down after just 10 months, but you are going to feel better when you have let go just 10 lbs or 20 lbs. Remember that you are not going to see yourself on a diet. You are adopting a long-term approach to letting go of the weight. We are trained to rush from one place to another, one project to another. So often we seem to travel at warp speed and we feel obliged to race towards any goal we set. But slow and steady often gets just the results you want. Approach your journey as a marathon, not a sprint, and you will be able to go the distance.

You are on a Journey for Life, the rest of your life. Enjoy the journey and take it nice and easy.

"

"Slow but steady
wins the race."

———

AESOP

"

S IS FOR SLEEP

Research shows that sleep loss can increase hunger and affect your body's metabolism in a way that makes weight loss more difficult. The average night's sleep has dropped from 10 hours (before the invention of the light bulb) to 6.9 hours. Prior to electricity, candles were blown out early in the evening and we slept more. And, of course, lack of sleep is now exacerbated by world-wide social media, TV, video games and irregular working hours.

Due to our busy lifestyle, many of us feel the one thing we can cut back on in order to get through the things we need to do, is sleep. However, remember that a good night's sleep may actually increase your productivity throughout the day because you have more energy, move about more and are able to think more clearly. Sleep deprivation affects memory, mood, weight gain and appetite.

There are mixed opinions on whether you should have something to eat before you go to sleep. I believe that you should not go to bed hungry. So, if you really feel that you are physically hungry and need a snack before bedtime make it light and low in protein. Protein makes your body think it should be active and could keep you awake.

For some people loss of sleep is a result of already being overweight and they suffer from sleep apnea, lower back pain and anxiety. A 16-year study at Harvard found that those who slept five hours or less were 32 times more likely to increase their weight than those who slept a minimum of seven hours per night.

"Sleep is the golden chain that ties health and our bodies together."

———

THOMAS DEKKER

S IS FOR SABOTEURS

Who is trying to sabotage your efforts? You? Your spouse? Your friends? You may have one or some of them in your life. Look at yourself honestly and ask if you sabotage yourself. I have clients who say that they let go the pounds until they reach a certain weight and they cannot go any lower. They start to over indulge once again and the weight creeps up. This may be because of a different way of thinking... Do you think "Well I've done well so far so I can indulge. Am I really going to like myself when I'm slim? Will I still be me? Will my friends still like me?" Could you be a little afraid of any changes that being slim will bring?

A saboteur can also be the spouse, friend or family member who says, "You look fine just as you are, just have a cookie – one won't harm you." They may mean well; they want to reassure you that you are lovable and worthwhile just as you are. However, you have to decide whether to accept that you are perfectly fine just as you are and that you don't need or want that extra cookie, or if you are going to be persuaded to have that one more bite.

There may be the friend who says "Let's share a dessert" and when you refuse, they look sad and say "Oh, well I guess I won't have one then. I can't eat a whole one, I need you to share it with me." The answer to that is "You decide for yourself what you want. I'm just not in the mood for dessert."

What about the dear, well-meaning person who makes that favorite pie for you, because they know you love it and that it has always made you feel good? You may think they would feel rejected if their love offering were refused, but you can be tactful. You could say you are full but you will have some later, or have just one bite, unless you choose to have more, then tell them how wonderful it is and put the rest out of sight.

Just remember that you do not owe ANYONE your good health – not anyone. What is the best way to age successfully? It is being healthy, independent, vitally alive, happy and free! So, beware the saboteurs.

S IS FOR STRESS

One of the essential elements to shedding weight and keeping it off is to learn how to handle your stress. There are few, if any, of us who live totally stress-free lives. When you are stressed the levels of cortisol in the brain increase, which can cause you to crave comfort foods. It may seem that the comfort food helps you to deal with the stress, but only for a very limited time. Very soon you realize that you are still stressed because you have not dealt with the cause of the stress.

The comfort food you eat leads to an overproduction of insulin and your blood-sugar levels soon begin to drop. You feel tired and irritable, and as you may well know, you crave more comfort food. The circle goes on and you gain weight.

So, if you are feeling stressed, it is usually a signal from your body that you need to address in some way other than eating. One way to calm oneself is to breathe diaphragmatically. Breathe in slowly and evenly through the nostrils. Become aware of how the abdomen expands, then the rib cage, then the entire lungs. To exhale, simply reverse the process. Do not strain. Never breathe beyond your capacity, trying to force air into the lungs. Just breathe rhythmically and easily. Self-hypnosis, another very useful tool for dealing with stress, can be taught by a qualified hypnotherapist and could serve you well in this instance.

T IS FOR THINK BEFORE YOU DRINK

It is being said that we are drinking ourselves into obesity. A University of North Carolina study found that Americans consume 450 calories a day from beverages, nearly twice as many as we did 30 years ago. Yes, you may want that occasional glass of wine and there are benefits to that, but too much alcohol just makes your efforts to be slim more difficult. When your body is busy processing alcohol it is not processing food or fat.

There is a lot written about diet sodas and the more I learn the more I recommend cutting them out altogether. There are ingredients in diet sodas that can, and usually do, increase your appetite. Regular soda contains an extraordinary amount of sugar. So, if you like the fizz you can drink sparkling water with a slice of lemon or orange in it.

When you visit the coffee shop, decide if that whipped topping really gives you value for the calories you consume.

I really enjoy beverages
that support my
good health

T IS FOR TRY

What are you thinking as you read this book? "Well, I'll give it a try. I've tried so many times before. I could try to lose the weight but I wonder if I can do it." How many times has one of those thoughts run through your mind? Well the more you try, the more you will go on doing just that – you will try.

Do you think that Sir Edmund Hillary thought "I think I'll try to conquer Mount Everest"? No, he didn't try, he set out to do it. Do you think Amelia Earhart thought "Let me try to cross the Atlantic, solo."? No, she set out to just do it. Eliminate the word try from your mental vocabulary. Don't even think about trying to reduce weight – just do it.

"When you do something for 6 weeks it becomes a habit. When you do it for 3 months it becomes a way of life."

———

ANONYMOUS

T IS FOR TO-GO BOX

Eating out is a national past-time. Portions are large. A client left my office and went to a national chain restaurant and ordered pasta. Her boyfriend wondered what she was doing as she moved her clenched fist along the side of the plate, measuring how many portions of pasta were on that plate. She had been served almost four portions of pasta. Before she became mindful of what she ate and how much she ate, she would have cleaned her plate.

Next time you go to a restaurant, order your to-go box so that it is delivered at the same time as you get your food. Then cut your food in half, put one half in the box, seal it and set it aside. The other half is your lunch/dinner and it will be much closer to the amount you need to eat. When you have left-overs to take home it is so tempting, while sitting there talking and waiting for the to-go box, to have just one more bite, and one more bite and suddenly it's not worth taking home what's left, so why not finish it up. Put the temptation in the to-go box at the beginning of the meal. It works!

T IS FOR TAKE TIME

Take time for yourself. Take time to **take care** of yourself. If you find yourself overwhelmed and stressing out, take some time out and do something that nourishes you, something that does not involve eating.

Life is busy, most people have many priorities and it is easy to put yourself last on the list. A basic advice for the self-employed is to pay yourself first or you may pay everything else and never have anything left for you. That is a rule that many do not adhere to when it comes to nourishing themselves. Find those few minutes to just let go, dream, relax, re-group. Take a long, long shower, or lie back in a silky bubble bath. Curl up in a big chair, in a robe and close your eyes for a moment or two. Take a short stroll in the summer sun. Plant a garden, a window-box, or sit and gaze at the sunset. Turn off the cell phone and be out of reach! The world will not come to an end in the 15 to 30 minutes that you are unavailable.

Ignoring your needs by putting them at the bottom of the priority list doesn't mean that they will just disappear, but it will likely mean that you will try to ignore them and reach for comfort food. It may seem the easiest and quickest way to nourish yourself but, of course, that is far from the truth. You will most likely be sabotaging any efforts you are making to live a healthy and balanced life. All too often we forget that we are human "beings", not human "doings", so allow yourself to just be.

Take time... make time... for yourself. Put yourself high on the list. Just a few minutes of me-time a day can make a tremendous difference to your well-being and success in reaching your goal.

U IS FOR USE YOUR SUBCONSCIOUS POWER

You have a very powerful resource in your subconscious mind. In your subconscious mind are stored all the memories, emotions, ideas and beliefs that you have accumulated throughout your life.

Comments may have been made to you about your weight that you have forgotten consciously, but they remain in the subconscious and may well be affecting the way you relate to food, the way you eat. For example, when I asked a client if she could see any benefit at all to keeping on her excess weight she thought for a moment and said, "Well my mother always told me that in the event of a disaster I would have more fat to keep me going than a thin person, so I would survive longer." So, each time she tried to shed weight her subconscious felt that she was becoming vulnerable and she would stop letting go of the weight. I suggested that perhaps, in the event of a disaster, a slender, healthy person might be able to get away from it, whereas an overweight person could not. Or maybe, if trapped in a confined space, the thin person could crawl out through a hole whereas the overweight person could not. We worked on that and she realized that it was quite safe to release the extra pounds.

Another person remembered her father saying "Men don't like skinny women. They like women with some meat on their bones." When her father told her that, it may have been so, but now that it is fashionable to be slim, she was in conflict. She wanted a love relationship but could not let go of that weight. Each time she reduced weight the subconscious thought would be "Men don't like skinny women." So, she had inner conflict because on the one hand she felt that she would be unattractive until she had become slim. On the other hand, she thought men would not be attracted to her if she was slim. She was frustrated and unhappy. We worked on her subconscious belief, but I encouraged her to think kindly of herself whatever her weight. To see herself for the very lovely young lady that she was, but to continue on the path to health and slenderness.

U IS FOR UNDERMINE

Beware the tendency to undermine yourself and your efforts. A client recently came to me after her first ten days of changing her eating habits. She said that she had done everything she felt she should do: she was eating less, she was more mindful of what she ate, she had no desire for sweet sugary food, and she had exercised more. She was four pounds down on the scale and her first reaction? Oh, that must be water. I asked her why she could not accept credit for doing things well and why did she not trust herself or the program.

Trust yourself, don't undermine your capabilities, your successes. If you are doing everything you need to be successful in reaching your goal, why not give yourself credit? Would you undermine your friend if they were successful in achieving their goal? No, you would congratulate them, so why undermine yourself and your efforts.

I give myself credit for
the positive changes
I see in my
eating habits

U IS FOR ULTIMATE GOAL

Stay aware of your ultimate goal – health, vitality and freedom. Yes, of course you want to be slim and strong but if you really examine what you want, don't you want to be the best you that you can be? If so, what does that mean to you?

What is your ultimate goal? You probably want to look good and feel good about yourself. You probably want to be healthy and free to have fun, do things with less effort, aspire to do the impossible.

Take time to think about your ultimate goal, what it is that you really want out of life? If you need a healthy body to help achieve your ultimate goal in life, start right now, not next week, not next month, start right now taking control and march resolutely towards your ultimate goal.

"If you don't know where you are going, you will probably end up somewhere else."

———

YOGI BERRA

V IS FOR VITAMINS

Much of today's food is highly processed, some is genetically engineered and research has shown that we do not get the same nutrition from our produce as we did in the past. While we can get some nutrition from the food we eat, in many instances we need to take vitamins to make up the deficit in our diet. First of all, you **must** speak with your doctor or nutritionist before embarking on a regimen of vitamins, especially if you are on medication. Some vitamins can negate the effects of medication or intensify its effect, neither of which will serve you well.

Over the years I have taken Vitamin C, as the body cannot store it, Vitamin B6 and B12 as they help the nervous system and Vitamin D as this affects our body in so many ways. Vitamin D is particularly needed if you live in an area that gets little sun. Each day more evidence is emerging that shows that Vitamin D may play a major role in keeping your brain sharp as you age.

Researchers at the University of Minnesota found that adequate Vitamin D levels in the body at the start of a low-calorie diet predict weight loss success, suggesting a possible role for Vitamin D in weight loss. Vitamin D is probably linked to maintaining a healthy body weight, according to research carried out at the Medical College of Georgia, USA.

There are, of course, other vitamins that can contribute to your good health **but always consult a nutritionist or doctor before you take any vitamins.**

V IS FOR VEGETABLES

Ah, vegetables! So many of us remember our parents insisting "You must eat your vegetables." Then perhaps came the resistance, and many times that resistance has lasted way into adulthood.

Vegetables are fabulous! Of course, there are various kinds, with different nutritional value. Potatoes and corn for example have lots of starch that converts into sugar and should be eaten in very small quantities. The rule of thumb is that the more color there is in a vegetable and the fresher and more leafy it is, the better. The FDA recommends at least five servings of fruit and vegetables a day. Find the vegetables that you really like, for then you will find it easier to eat your daily quota. Remember, eating healthy does not mean you have to eat food you don't like! Also be aware that all vegetables are not created equal so sitting down every day to five servings of white potatoes is not what it's about. Variety is the key so find those vegetables that you like and enjoy!

W IS FOR WATER, WONDERFUL WATER

Water – the best kept secret weapon. Most of our body is made up of water. 80% of our blood, 73% of our brain, 79% of muscle and up to 30% of bone is water.

About 75% of Americans are chronically dehydrated. Most people do not realize that they are dehydrated. Signs of dehydration are thirst, fatigue, headache and decrease in urination. Just a 2% drop in body water can trigger fuzzy short-term memory, and loss of focus and concentration. Water is excellent for the skin. See the difference when your body is adequately hydrated.

For decades eight 8oz glasses of water per day has been the recommended intake. However, this is a suggestion and you can learn to know your body and recognize its needs. It is possible, if you are healthy, that your body needs less than this, five or six glasses seems to work well for some people, especially if they are eating a diet containing vegetables and fruits that are high in water content.

Before reaching for a pill if you have a headache, drink a large glass of water. Before having that snack, drink a large glass of water and then decide if you still need the snack. In many instances you were thirsty, not hungry.

Drinking a large glass of water 10 – 15 minutes before a meal helps you to feel satisfied more quickly and helps your food to digest properly. It aids your elimination system to function properly to cleanse waste products and waste materials out of your body in an easy, natural way. Water keeps your kidneys healthy. W is for water – Wonderful Water!

W IS FOR WHOLE GRAINS

Whole grains are sometimes referred to as "the Staff of Life" and have been the staple food of almost all civilization throughout history. Whole grains should be the very basis of your eating regimen. However, if you are **diabetic**, consult with a nutritionist or dietician.

Americans eat only 1% of whole grains in their daily diet. The grains we eat are mostly refined. We eat white bread, white pasta, white rice, and white flour. Whole grains such as barley, corn, rye, oats, quinoa and millet should be included in your eating plan.

Beans and legumes are closely related to whole grains and are of great benefit. They are a wonderful low-fat, high-protein food full of nutrition and are an excellent source of fiber.

Whole grains are easy to cook and easy to use. Make a pot of whole grains and beans at the weekend, rinse well and store in your fridge. You can add them to salads or have with protein and vegetables throughout the week. Get into the habit of making whole grains part of your daily diet. You will be so glad you did!

W IS FOR WISH LIST

Do you have a Wish List? Do you find yourself saying "Oh, how I wish I had… I wish I could…"? When clients come to me, I ask them to leave their wish list behind. They may come in with a wish list but I ask them to leave with a "To Do" list.

How does your Wish List go? Oh, I wish I had the willpower to stop snacking in the evening. I wish I could stop eating candy. I wish I were able to… I'm sure you can fill in the blank. Very often the wish is followed with… but, as in "I wish I had the willpower to stop snacking in the evening *but* I don't. I wish I could stop eating candy *but* I can't."

The To Do List would have the word *and* instead of *but*. I have the willpower to stop snacking in the evening, *and* I will do so. I can stop eating candy *and* I am going to.

"I've wished for things and never really had the chance. It's time to stop dreaming and do something about it. You've got to know what you want, then…go."

———

DEB CALETTI, THE SIX RULES OF MAYBE

W IS FOR WEIGH-IN

How often do you weigh yourself? Weighing is a choice. If you choose to weigh in, do so no more than once a week, preferably on the same day at the same time and in the same state of dress or undress. It is a good idea to put your scale in a cupboard, out of sight, and not right next to the shower, to discourage the habit of just getting on to see what you weigh after your daily shower.

I had a client who said "I am absolutely sick and tired of thinking about food. It consumes my thoughts all day." During our interview I asked how often she weighed herself. "Every morning,' she said, "as soon as I have showered, I step on the scale. I need to see if I am a pound up or down and then eat accordingly." I explained that in doing that she was putting herself in the arena where she had to think about food all day long. If she was up an ounce or two, she would think about what she couldn't eat and if she was down an ounce or two, she rewarded herself.

I have another client who never jumps on the scale. She has shed more than 90 lbs by going about her life, eating when she is hungry, choosing carefully the foods she eats, but not depriving herself. She is loving her renewed energy, feeling fit and healthy and feeling good about the way her clothes look and feel on her.

Remember that muscle is denser than fat and sometimes it is through the fit of our clothing that we see the change in shape and weight. Ideally, weekly weight reduction should be 1% of your total body weight.

It was never intended that we become consumed by food – we are meant to consume food! There are so many other things to think about during the day that food should not be the main focus of every day. So, weigh in occasionally and then forget about the scale.

W IS FOR WASTE NOT, WANT NOT

Ah, haven't we all heard that at some time? We are conditioned not to waste, so when we see that small amount of food left on the plate it seems wrong to throw it away – that is good food! However, I would like to suggest you see waste in a different light. When you are satisfied with what you have eaten it is time to stop eating. That's it – STOP. If you eat that extra food because you feel it is wrong to throw it out, think on the following: When you eat unneeded food three things happen.

- Your organs that have worked efficiently for you are now asked to overwork. You place a strain on all your internal organs.
- Some of that extra food goes on the waist, and is stored in other parts of the body.
- That which is left goes through the intestines and is released as – waste. Yes, that food still becomes waste but it is toxic waste. Chemicals are needed to deal with it. Our oceans are becoming more and more polluted, some of which is attributed to sewage. You may have seen beaches closed because of sewage spills into the ocean. It is far better for your body and for the planet to throw out the uneaten food. It will re-cycle more easily and naturally.

Change your thinking. It is a responsible act to throw out excess, unwanted food. It is a responsible act for your body and for the planet.

X IS FOR XYLITOL

What is that? Xylitol is a natural sweetener that comes from fruits and vegetables and also from the birch tree. While Xylitol is as sweet as table sugar (sucrose) it has about 40% fewer calories and 75% fewer carbohydrates, making it a low-calorie alternative to table sugar. Absorbed more slowly than sugar, it does not contribute to high blood sugar levels or the resulting hyperglycemia caused by insufficient insulin response.

There are, of course, other natural sweeteners but if you have an intolerance to any of them and do not wish to use sugar, you may want to explore the use of Xylitol.

PLEASE NOTE: As with any new food choice, speak with your doctor before taking Xylitol as there are possible side effects.

Y IS FOR YOU CAN DO IT

There is a good chance that you have reduced weight before. Once the subconscious mind knows that it can be done, it also knows that it can be done again. One good example is that of a person being able to swim the English Channel, a waterway 21 miles wide, between England and France. It was considered impossible until Matthew Webb of the UK succeeded on August 25 1875. Following that, others were successful and in 1926 an American woman, Gertrude Ederle was the first female to successfully swim the Channel. Why were these people now able to do something previously considered impossible? Because they knew it could be done!

So many of my clients say they know what they should be doing. They just need help doing it. That is why they come to me for hypnosis.

You really are the writer, actor, editor and producer in your play of life. At times it may seem as if this is not so, but remember that you always have a choice, so many times you can choose how a scene plays out. This especially applies to what you eat, when you eat and how much you eat. When you "make up your mind" you can do it. Think of the many things you have decided to do in the past. Now think of how you did them. You can do it!

"Whether you think you can, or think you can't, you're right."

———

ATTRIBUTED TO HENRY FORD

Y IS FOR YESTERDAY

You've heard it before: yesterday is past, the future is unknown, all we have is the present. Today really is the first day of the rest of your life. So, put yesterday behind you, you will never have it again. What is done is done, what has gone, has gone.

Now is the moment. Seize it! You are making choices right now. Don't live in yesterday. What you did then, what you thought then, was… then. It was a different time and different you.

Let yesterday be where it belongs, in the past.

"Don't let yesterday
use up too much
of today."

———

WILL ROGERS

Y IS FOR YOGA

Yoga is a gentle way of moving, of stretching the body. When you are letting go of that unwanted weight you will want to move your body as much as possible. If you are very overweight the process needs to be as gentle as possible and yoga has many health benefits, as well as aiding the loss of weight. It strengthens muscles, stretches the body and calms the mind.

If you do not want to go to a class, there are some excellent downloads you can buy and online videos and lessons that you can do in the privacy of your own home. Take it easy and go only as far as you are comfortable. Should you feel discomfort stop immediately. As with any form of exercise it is advisable to speak with your health provider before trying something new. Then just relax, listen to the calming background music and gently stretch. It feels good!

Z IS FOR ZONE OUT

In today's world we so often feel the need to be rushing here and there, dealing with this and that, achieving something or another. Do you take time to stop and smell the roses – or the strawberries? Don't forget that a whiff of strawberries can increase your metabolism! You're not in a race, you are just on a voyage through life. Is every day spent in stormy waters or can you allow yourself a little calm sailing? Try to find a few moments, perhaps first thing in the morning, or during a lunch break to just zone out.

It's not easy to think of nothing, and if you can't do that just let yourself drift into a sweet place of reverie. Feel yourself smile as you bring forth a pleasant memory. Everybody must be able to find one thing that makes them smile. It may be from long ago, something you've tucked away at the back of your mind. So, find it in that quiet moment. Feel that feeling of well-being, put aside the doubts and fears and have the moment. Think perhaps of the Zen story of the man with the strawberry. He found a moment of bliss – you can too.

Z IS FOR ZEST FOR LIFE

Do you have it? Do you have a zest for life? Are you going to arrive at the Golden Gates excited, disheveled, whooping and hollering "WOW, what a ride!" Or are you going to limp in full of regret for the things left undone, the good you let pass you by?

This is the time. Make a change! Give yourself the gift of joy. Dream, dream big, not just about the new slim, vital you, but about your life!

Enjoy it!

"Go confidently in the direction of your dreams! Live the life you've imagined."

—

HENRY DAVID THOREAU

CONCLUSION

My goal in writing this book has been to offer suggestions and food for thought that have been helpful to my clients over the years I have been working with them, as they became slimmer and fitter. My hope is that you will find the information helpful to you as you continue on your journey to living life easily in a lighter, healthier body, and experiencing the freedom that comes with it.

If you have any questions I invite you to visit my website www.hazelnewsom.com. I would love to hear from you.

ENJOY YOUR JOURNEY

Printed in the United States
by Baker & Taylor Publisher Services